I0123332

Degenerative Disc Disease Explained

Facts & Information

Including treatment, surgery, symptoms, exercises, causes, physical therapy, neck, back pain, and much more!

By: Frederick Earlstein

Copyrights and Trademarks

All rights reserved. No part of this book may be reproduced or transformed in any form or by any means, graphic, electronic, or mechanical, including photocopying, recording, taping, or by any information storage retrieval system, without the written permission of the author.

This publication is Copyright © 2013. All products, graphics, publications, software and services mentioned and recommended in this publication are protected by trademarks. In such instance, all trademarks & copyright belong to the respective owners.

Disclaimer and Legal Notice

This product is not legal, medical, or accounting advice and should not be interpreted in that manner. You need to do your own due-diligence to determine if the content of this product is right for you. While every attempt has been made to verify the information shared in this publication, neither the author, neither publisher, nor the affiliates assume any responsibility for errors, omissions or contrary interpretation of the subject matter herein. Any perceived slights to any specific person(s) or organization(s) are purely unintentional.

We have no control over the nature, content and availability of the web sites listed in this book. The inclusion of any web site links does not necessarily imply a recommendation or endorse the views expressed within them. We take no responsibility for, and will not be liable for, the websites being temporarily unavailable or being removed from the internet.

The accuracy and completeness of information provided herein and opinions stated herein are not guaranteed or warranted to produce any particular results, and the advice and strategies, contained herein may not be suitable for every individual. Neither the author nor the publisher shall be liable for any loss incurred as a consequence of the use and application, directly or indirectly, of any information presented in this work. This publication is designed to provide information in regard to the subject matter covered.

Neither the author nor the publisher assume any responsibility for any errors or omissions, nor do they represent or warrant that the ideas, information, actions, plans, suggestions contained in this book is in all cases accurate. It is the reader's responsibility to find advice before putting anything written in this book into practice. The information in this book is not intended to serve as legal, medical, or accounting advice.

Foreword

Any of us who survived high school biology class are at least vaguely aware of how the human spine looks. Perhaps your classroom had the ubiquitous skeleton dangling from a hook on a rolling stand like mine did.

In my high school, his name was Melvin, and his bones were well travelled. At Halloween he showed up in the principle's leather desk chair, and at one homecoming pep rally, Melvin was present in the gym wearing a sign that read, "Oldest living graduate."

The popular rumor at the time was that Melvin was a real skeleton, the remains of some ancient biology teacher who more or less desiccated away in his chair grading papers.

Over the past few years, as I've dealt with episodic neck pain from degenerative disc disease, I've thought about Melvin a great deal. I do remember having to pass a quiz that called for each of us to march up to the front of the classroom and identify at least 15 of his prominent bones.

Until my neck started hurting, however, I had absolutely no appreciation for the marvel of engineering that is the human spine.

I've watched my dog push out his front paws, elevate his backside, and give his own backbone a thorough stretch and wondered if our prehistoric ancestors did us any favors when they stood up for the first time.

Foreword

On my first visit to the doctor, I was informed that my neck pain was an aspect of getting older. I didn't enjoy hearing that any more than I liked the young optometrist who prescribed my bifocals saying, "As we age, our eyes change . . ."

What really annoyed me about my neck pain was the fact that many of my friends who are of the same "vintage" as myself were not experiencing the same thing. After working with a physical therapist, however, I realized that many of my unconscious habits were the real root of my problem.

Chances are very good that all of my friends have just as much degenerative disc disease as I have, but they do a better job of maintaining their weight, taking moderate exercise, staying well hydrated, and putting down the cigarettes.

I had to make some definite lifestyle changes in order to be pain free. I even had to learn how to pick up objects the right way, and get a pillow that supported my head at night rather than making my neck pain worse.

At first, I was not a willing patient. I wanted a pill to make it all go away. I didn't want to have to go to physical therapy. At one point, in great frustration, I asked my doctor, "Why can't you just give me a new disc?"

Foreword

He made me watch a video of a cervical disc replacement surgery. I quit protesting, went to physical therapy, and ordered the expensive memory foam pillow he recommended. When I took responsibility for my role in aggravating my neck issues, I was able to address them effectively with conservative treatment.

Casually at first, and then with growing interest, I began to read about spinal health. It was a time-consuming process, one that involved keeping a dictionary open on my desk to sort out the medical terms I was encountering.

By the time my neck was once again moving as it should, I decided to compile my research into this book. The bad news is that degenerative disc disease is, indeed, a consequence of aging, and its effects are not just confined to the neck as they were in my case.

You may well be one of the many people suffering from lower back pain seeking to understand and correct your problem. It's also possible, though rarer, for degenerative disc disease to affect the mid- to upper back.

The good news in all these cases, however, is that it is possible to have the degeneration and be pain free. There are many viable options for managing the condition offered by both conventional and alternative medicine. Unfortunately, there are times, however, when surgery is the only option.

Foreword

It is my hope that this text will help you to more fully understand your degenerative disc problem and to make the best and most informed decisions you can about how to address it.

Back in the day, Melvin the Biology Room Skeleton was, in fact, revealing to my eyes the intricacies of the human spine. If I had appreciated that fact, I might have taken better precautions to preserve my spinal health.

I discovered through personal experience that it's never too late to start taking better care of our bodies – and our bones, in particular some highly specialized bones called intervertebral discs.

Read on to find out why doing something as simple as drinking enough water every day can completely change your own spinal health.

Acknowledgments

I would like to express my gratitude towards my family, friends, and colleagues for their kind co-operation and encouragement which helped me in completion of this book.

My thanks and appreciations go to my colleagues and people who have willingly helped me out with their abilities.

Acknowledgments

Table of Contents

Table of Contents

Table of Contents

Table of Contents

Part 1 – Disc Disease Overview

The phrase "disc disease" is misleading. This condition is a natural consequence of aging. The degeneration refers to alterations in the composition and function of the spinal cartilage, not necessarily to a progressive worsening of the accompanying symptoms.

When degenerative disc disease (DDD) is actively symptomatic, the problems it causes are typically located in the neck and/or lower back. The condition is highly variable in nature.

In some cases, the individual is completely unaware of its presence, and in others symptoms may actually improve depending on how the problem is addressed.

The Structure of the Human Spine

The spinal column is responsible for keeping humans upright, and is the center of our skeletal system. The length of the spine varies by height, but on average it will be 28 inches (71 cm) in men and 24 inches (61 cm) in women.

The Spinal Vertebrae

A total of 26 bony "blocks" or vertebrae separated by cushioning discs form the structure of the spine, which is divided into distinct regions:

Part 1 – Disc Disease Overview

- The cervical region or neck is composed of seven vertebrae. It is the most flexible portion of the spine.

- The thoracic region or mid-back includes 12 vertebrae.

- The lumbar region, or lower back, involves five vertebrae.

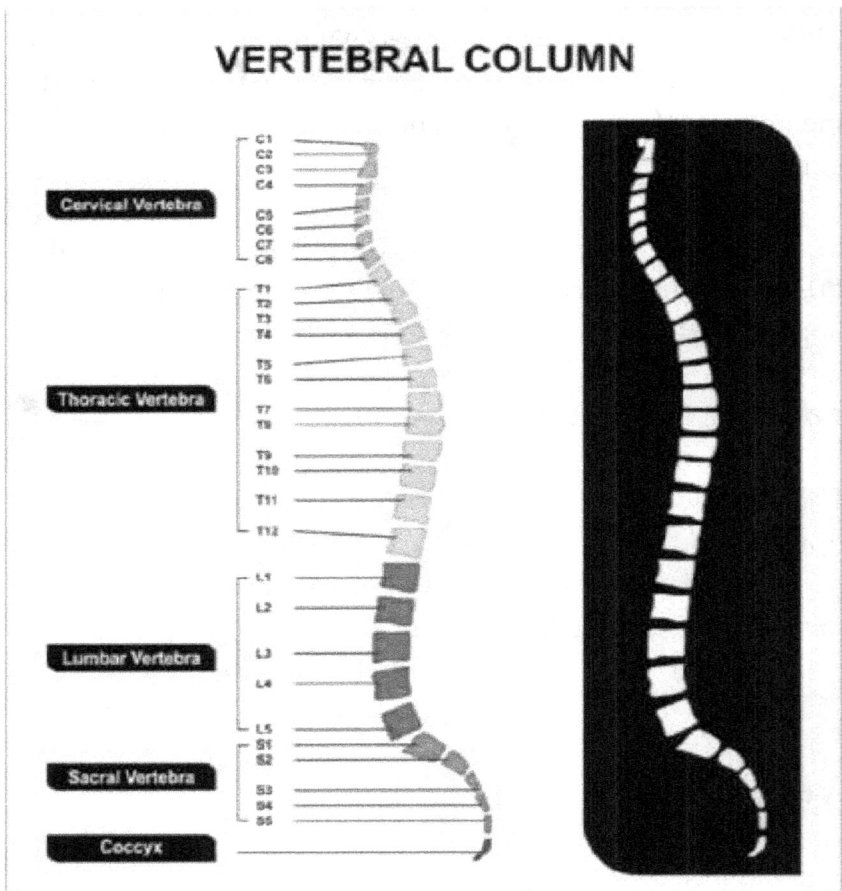

VERTEBRAL COLUMN

Cervical Vertebra — C1, C2, C3, C4, C5, C6, C7, C8

Thoracic Vertebra — T1, T2, T3, T4, T5, T6, T7, T8, T9, T10, T11, T12

Lumbar Vertebra — L1, L2, L3, L4, L5

Sacral Vertebra — S1, S2, S3, S4, S5

Coccyx

Below the last lumbar vertebrae, there are five more sacral vertebrae fused into the sacrum bone that run to the mid-buttock region of the body. Below that, lies the coccyx or tailbone. These are the least flexible portions of the overall structure.

If you were to view the spine from the side, it does not make a straight line, but rather follows four curves. The neck (cervical) and lower back (lumbar) portions curve inward, while the upper back (thoracic) and base (sacral) curve outward.

The curves stabilize and strengthen the total spine and help humans to remain balanced in our upright, standing position. The vertebrae grow larger toward the base of the spine because there they carry more weight.

The Function of the Discs

There are 23 discs that lie between the vertebrae that are designed to act as cushions, minimizing the impact of our daily movements on the spinal column. These structures also allow the spine to rotate and to move sideways.

There are no discs present between the skull and the first vertebra, or between the first and second vertebrae themselves.

Often you will see the discs compared to jelly donuts because they have a soft center called the nucleus pulposus. Each disc is a cartilaginous joint that compresses and decompresses (becomes thinner and thicker) as pressure is applied to it throughout the day.

At night, the discs get a chance to rest. Humans will always be slightly taller if measured in the morning than in the evening by a variation of about 1.5-2 cm.

An outer ring, the annulus fibrosus, which is comprised of ligaments, keeps the soft inner core contained so it can serve as a shock absorber.

The Spinal Cord

The spinal cord is encased in the center of the spine for protection. Each vertebra incorporates structures that allow spinal nerves to exit out of the spinal canal and branch outward.

These spinal nerves are responsible for carrying signals from the brain to the muscles and internal organs, and for relaying back sensory information gathered in the body.

This includes the ability to:

- feel heat and cold
- sense vibrations
- distinguish dull and sharp sensations
- sense the position of the limbs (arms and legs)

Additionally, the spinal cord plays a key role in the regulation of blood pressure, heart rate, and body temperature.

If these nerves are damaged, the effect can be extensive. Injuries to the cervical nerves (C1-C8) can result in quadriplegia, affecting the movement of the arms, hands, and legs. Damage to the thoracic nerves (T1-T12) may cause paraplegia, affecting the motion of the legs.

This complex interaction of the brain, spinal cord, and spinal nerves forms the body's central nervous system. Often the symptoms of degenerative disc disease include neurological deficits like tingling in the extremities when some of these nerves become compressed.

When Degeneration Sets In

As humans age, the discs that separate the spinal vertebrae change in composition and size, leading to greater curvature of the spine. This explains why we become shorter as we get older.

Inflammatory Disc Pain

The principle alteration in the structure of the discs involves protein and water. As both are lost, the discs thin and weaken, losing their flexibility. These diminished capacities make the discs less effective as shock absorbers.

Discs have no way to repair themselves because they do not have their own blood supply. In fact, the discs don't have many nerve endings, but the adjacent annulus fibrous does.

The proteins that leak out of the interior of the disc are inflammatory in nature, and are thus responsible for one type of pain that accompanies the degenerative process. The pain can also be mechanical, however.

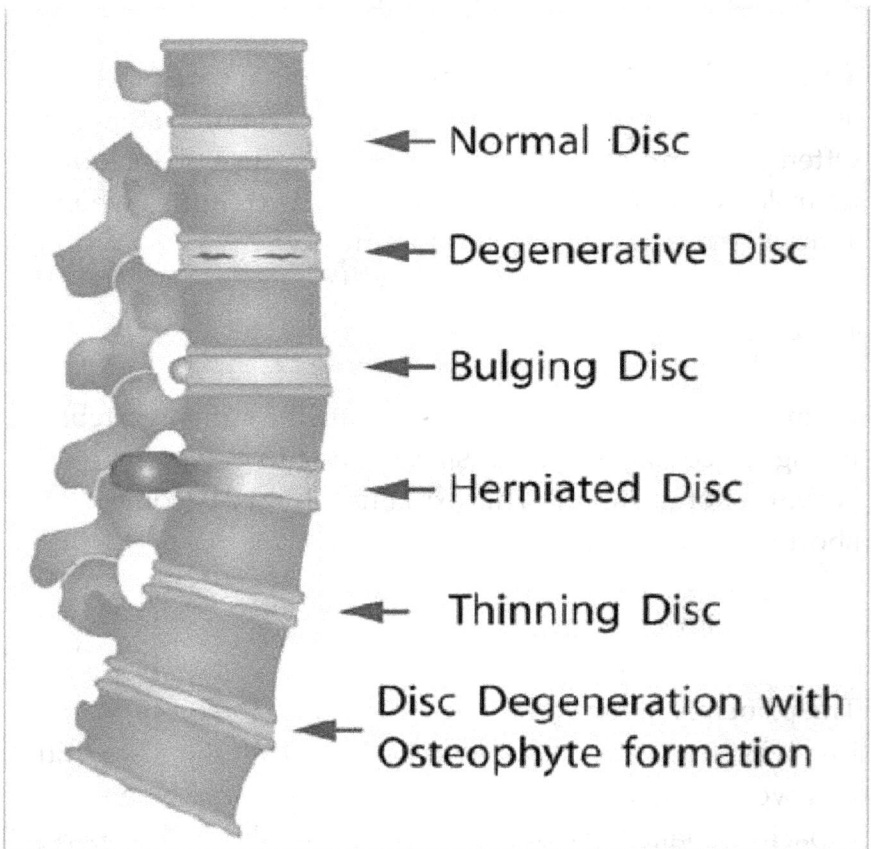

← Normal Disc

← Degenerative Disc

← Bulging Disc

← Herniated Disc

← Thinning Disc

← Disc Degeneration with Osteophyte formation

Part 1 – Disc Disease Overview

Mechanical Disc Pain

When disc pain is mechanical, a nerve root is being physically compressed, typically as a result of a herniation due to tears in the annulus.
The disc's inner "jelly" gets forced outward, causing the disc to bulge (herniate) and sometimes to rupture. If enough fluid leaks out of the center of the disc, it may collapse.

The more the distance between the vertebrae shrinks, the less the bones are cushioned from the impact of movement and the less flexible they become.

Spinal Stenosis

The collapse and decompression of the spine can lead to spinal stenosis. This narrowing of the spine's open spaces puts further pressure on the spinal cord and nerves, and happens most commonly in the neck and lower back.

Additionally, the facet joints located between and behind the vertebrae for stabilization may begin to shift. Normally, these joints are in almost constant motion, but with spinal decompression, the bone may begin to overgrow leading to the development of bone spurs.

Bone Spurs

Bone spurs or osteophytes are the body's attempts to stop excessive and painful spinal motion, but if the spurs grow into the spinal canal, they begin to press on the nerves causing even more pain.

Thus, the degeneration that begins with water loss in the joints can move through a progressive alteration of healthy spinal function with a cascading set of painful symptoms.

Exacerbating factors in this progression include, but are not limited to:

- being overweight
- having poor posture
- lifting heavy objects on a regular basis
- being subject to repetitive motion
- smoking

Generally, the progression of degenerative disc disease is so slow people don't realize the discs in their spines are changing. Rarely is the condition so severe as to require surgery.

On the other end of the spectrum, however, pain may be sufficiently debilitating to limit daily activities. This pain may present in the lower back or neck, but can also radiate into the shoulders, arms, buttocks, and legs. Twisting and reaching upward typically make the discomfort worse.

Part 1 – Disc Disease Overview

Diagnosing Degenerative Disc Disease

A diagnosis of degenerative disc disease starts with an extensive medical history. This will include questions about:

- symptoms (past and present)
- the pattern of change in those symptoms
- past injuries or illnesses
- treatment or intervention for past illnesses and injuries
- descriptions of current and past activities

During the course of the examination, the doctor will test for range of motion and look for areas up and down the spine that are tender or that are exhibiting nerve-related damage.

There will also be an assessment of sensations in other areas of the body to detect the presence of:

- tingling or a "pins and needles" feeling
- any numbness that may be present
- weaknesses and diminished reflexes

Other conditions like infections, tumors, fractures, strains, and muscle injuries will be ruled out, often by the use of imaging tests including X-rays and MRIs.

When a determination of degenerative disc disease is made, courses of treatment and intervention will be discussed.

Strategies to cope with disc disease always begin with a conservative approach.

It's important to remember that flare-ups of disc pain are highly episodic and heavily influenced by the presence of inflammation in the body. Early treatment will focus on coping strategies and pain relief with an eye toward behaviour modification and exercise to prevent future incidents.

Only in rarely and unusually severe cases is surgery recommended for degenerative disc disease, and then only after all other avenues have been fully explored.

Special Section – Spinal Health Tips

Prevention is critical in managing the potentially painful cycle of degenerative disc disease. The American Chiropractic Association has formulated a set of recommendations for maintaining good spinal health, which includes the following points.

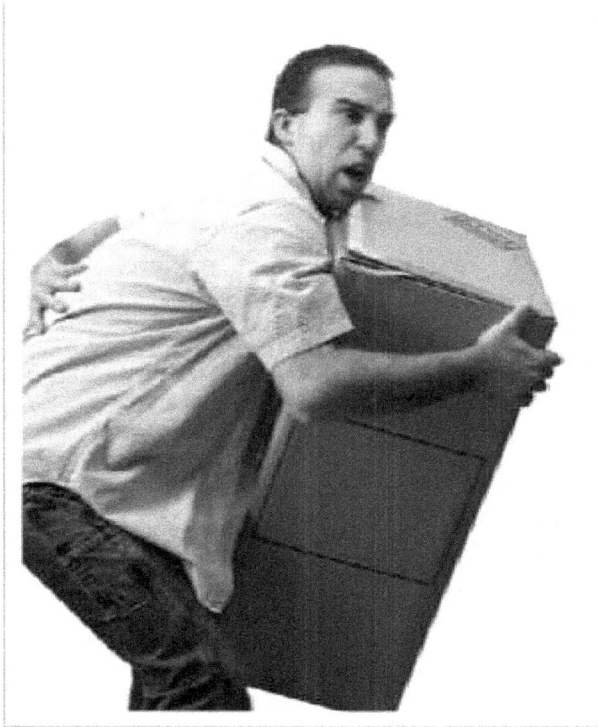

Practice Safe Lifting Techniques

The most dangerous movement you can make with a potential negative effect on the spine is twisting, but in combination with lifting, this action can be especially detrimental.

Remember with heavy items that pushing is easier than pulling. Use your legs to push rather than straining your upper body. If lifting the object is the only option, get some help.

Stand in a Supportive Way

The most supportive standing position is to keep one foot just a little in front of the other. Make sure your knees are bent slightly to relieve the pressure on your lower back.

Standing bent forward at the waist for extended periods of time will weaken the muscles of the lower back and intensify pain. Always avoid this position.

Sit With Proper Posture

Slouching while sitting will only aggravate any back pain you are experiencing. Instead, keep your knees somewhat higher than your hips.

Your back should be straight, but preserve the natural curvature of the lower back and sit with your head up.

Be Careful Reaching and Bending

If you have to reach for anything higher than the level of your shoulders, stand on a secure stool. Straining while reaching upward is harmful to your neck and mid-back.

This same motion can also create shoulder problems that will only further compromise your ability to use your back in a natural way.

To pick things up off a table or the floor, never bend down from the waist. Kneel on one knee and get as close to the item as possible. Keep your other foot flat on the floor and lift the item.

As an alternate technique, bend at the knees and hold the object close to your body. Use your legs to lift, not your back.

Carry Loads Wisely

Carry objects close to your body, especially if they are heavy. If you are carrying two small objects, distribute the weight evenly, carrying one in each hand.

Eat Well and Exercise

There's no way of getting around the fact that extra weight strains the spine. Stay within 10 lbs. / 4.45 kg of your ideal weight. Extra pounds around the waist are especially detrimental, placing extra strain on all the muscles, tendons, and ligaments of the lower back.

(Always consult your primary care physician before undertaking a program of exercise, no matter how moderate.)

Sleeping Is Hard Work!

If you sleep on your back, you're placing approximately 50 lbs. / 22.7 kg of pressure on your spine. If this is the only way you can fall asleep, keep a pillow under your knees to reduce the load on your back by as much as half.

A better position is to lie on your side with a pillow between your knees. Special pillows are available to support this position that you can anchor in place around one leg with self-attaching straps.

Listen to your body. Even if you are used to sleeping in one position, find what works to keep your spine from hurting and use it!

Give Up the Cigarettes

Studies prove that people who smoke experience more spine pain and recover more slowly from injuries. The effect of the nicotine keeps blood from flowing properly around the spine making healing more difficult.

Special Section – Spinal Health Tips

These guidelines are no guarantee that your back will be completely free of pain, but by learning to move, stand, sit, and sleep properly, you can reduce your chances of experiencing severe, prolonged pain.

Part 2 – Disc Disease by Region

Degenerative disc disease differs according to the region of the spine involved. The areas most commonly affected, in order of occurrence are:

- lumbar or lower back
- cervical or neck
- thoracic or mid-back

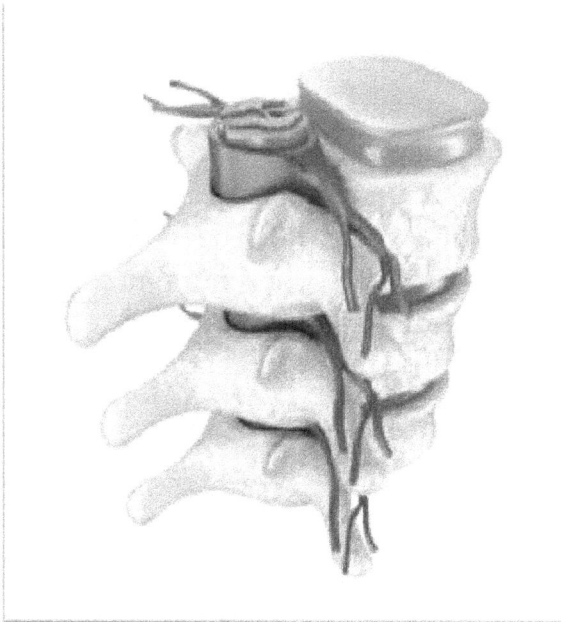

Whenever possible, the symptoms caused by degenerative disc disease are addressed conservatively, with surgery an option of last resort only.

For the purposes of this discussion, we will look at the effects of disc disease starting with the neck and moving down the spinal column.

Cervical Disc Disease

Medical research indicates that approximately 67% of the world's adult population will experience neck pain from cervical disc disease at some point in their lives.

Neck problems are especially common in later life due to accumulated damage to the vertebrae from decades of repetitive stress. Degenerative disc disease in the cervical region is more complicated than just experiencing pain, however.

Typically, as the discs in the neck begin to deteriorate, the person also suffers weakness and numbness in the shoulders, arms, and hands. This can lead to loss of flexibility and mobility that effects both work and leisure activities.

The Cervical Spine

The seven vertebrae of the cervical spine provide stability for the neck and allow for the smooth turning of the head. They support the least amount of weight, but are subject to greater stresses due to the extensive range of their mobility.

The vertebrae begin at the base of the skull and move downward to connect to the thoracic spine. They are designated as C1 through C7. The first vertebrae C1, forms a ring that rotates around C2.

Rotation, Flexion, Extension

The cervical vertebrae allow for rotation, flexion, and extension of the head and neck. Rotation is the movement of the head from side to side, which is primarily controlled by C1 and C2.

Flexion is the act of moving the head forward, while extension is the backward motion. This range is controlled by C5 through C7.

These basic motions, however, can occur in a huge range of sequences. Using our necks, we can look left and up, for instance, in a smooth curve.

Most of us give very little thought to just how smoothly these movements take place until they are interrupted. Then, when pain does surface, we are shocked at how much it affects our day-to-day lives.

Suddenly swiveling to check for oncoming traffic at a busy intersection is excruciating. However, if we don't execute that motion, we risk being involved in an accident.

Under such real-life circumstances, the seriousness of neck problems becomes all too readily apparent. It is for this reason that people are often desperate to correct their neck pain, and wrongly assume that surgery is their only option.

Part 2 – Disc Disease by Region

Prevalence of Neck Problems

While it is more common to see disc degeneration in the lumbar spine, neck pain runs lower back pain a close second in prevalence.

Under the age of 40, only about 25% of the population develops signs of degenerative issues in the neck. From age 40 and beyond, however, the number jumps to 60%. This includes pinched nerves and the formation of bone spurs.

Types of Neck Pain

There are varying types of neck pain. Not all forms are associated with disc degeneration, but can rather be attributed to soft tissue injuries to the muscles, ligaments, and tendons.

Common causes of these complaints are auto accidents that result in "whiplash," or getting a "crick" from sleeping the wrong way. Sometimes just carrying a heavy object will strain a neck muscle creating stiffness and soreness that can take as much as 2 weeks to resolve.

Pain that lasts from 2 weeks to a few months, however, is a sign that either a more serious injury has occurred, or that a degenerative disease is present. The common culprits are disc degeneration and arthritis, singularly or in combination.

Part 2 – Disc Disease by Region

Initial symptoms of neck problems of this type include loss of flexibility and stiffness or "tension" that is most often felt in the evenings.

Over time, the condition can continue to worsen until the discomfort migrates into the shoulders and arms. At this point, functional quality of life can be severely compromised.

Diagnosing Cervical Disc Disease

After taking a medical history and conducting a neurological exam, your doctor will measure your neck's extension, and evaluate its flexibility.

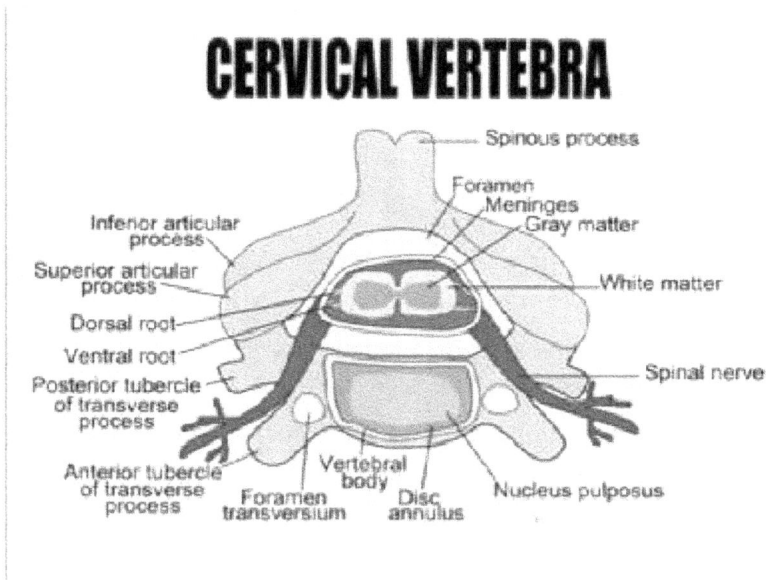

CERVICAL VERTEBRA

Imaging procedures may be required, such as X-rays, an MRI, or a CT scan. These tests allow for a visual inspection of the condition of the vertebrae and spinal cord to help identify the origin of the pain.

These imaging scans will also reveal the presence of any arthritis, which may exist as a separate condition or in conjunction with disc degeneration.

Treating Cervical Disc Disease

The first line of defense in the early stages of cervical disc disease addresses reducing both inflammation and pain. In most cases, only over-the-counter medications are required.

The best options are non-steroidal anti-inflammatory painkillers including:

- acetaminophen
- ibuprofen
- naproxen

If these drugs don't work, prescription steroids may be indicated. Some cases could require narcotic painkillers.

Regardless of the painkillers used, alternating applications of heat and ice can provide additional relief, and reduce how much medication has to be taken.

Physical therapy, including cervical traction and gentle manipulation are routinely used. Patients may work with a physical therapist, a chiropractor, a massage therapist, or some combination of all of these professionals.

Cervical collars and pillows are used to provide support during healing and are especially beneficial at night to improve the position of the head and neck. It is quite common for misalignment during sleep to exacerbate neck pain.

The overall goal of a complete therapy plan is to improve range of motion and posture while strengthening the supporting muscles of the neck. Cervical pain rarely remains constant throughout a person's life, tending to be more episodic in nature.

Conservative treatment for a flare up of neck pain should lead to improvement of the condition within six weeks. Rarely is surgery required, but when it is, the predominant procedure is a discectomy.

Cervical Discectomy or Fusion

In severe cases of cervical disc degeneration, the diseased disc will be removed and replaced with an artificial metal disc (cervical discectomy) or by cervical fusion.

(Both procedures will be discussed in Part 3, which considers Standard Medical Treatments.)

When surgery is indicated, the standard period of recovery is three months to one year, followed by changes in lifestyle and habits to keep the intact vertebrae of the cervical region healthier.

Typically this includes exercise, eating a good diet, and stopping smoking if tobacco use has been a factor.

Thoracic Disc Disease

Thoracic disc disease is much less common than cervical or lumbar issues, but when it is present, it causes pain in the upper or mid-back regions.

There are 12 vertebrae in this section, which is that portion of the spine below the neck connected to the ribs. It is fairly common for a disc in this region to become herniated, exerting pressure on nerve roots or the spinal cord.

Disc disease in the thoracic spine does not always result in pain, however. In a controlled study with 90 pain-free patients, 73% showed clear evidence of disc degeneration and herniation.

This may suggest that when back pain is present in the thoracic region, the real cause is some sort of trauma to the upper back rather than the aging of the disc themselves.

Such injuries might occur as the result of a fall, or as a consequence of playing some type of sport.

If the pressure on the spinal cord is significant, spinal cord dysfunction or myelopathy can result. Symptoms might then include poor balance, weakness in the legs, and bowel or bladder dysfunction.

Thoracic Disc Herniation

Thoracic disc herniation presents with one of three potential patterns of protrusion:

- central
- lateral
- centro-lateral

Symptoms will differ in each case.

- With a central protrusion, pain is in the upper back, with a potential for spinal cord dysfunction depending on the size of the herniation.

- In instances of lateral protrusion, exiting nerves are most typically affected, with chest wall and/or abdominal pain resulting.

- Centro-lateral protrusions present with a combination of upper back pain, chest and abdominal pain, and potential spinal cord dysfunctions.

Symptoms are always further delineated by the size and location of the disc.

Part 2 – Disc Disease by Region

Diagnosing Thoracic Disc Disease

Patients with problems in the thoracic spine report isolated and/or radiating pain in the upper back that may be worse when they cough or sneeze.

Since pain in this region may also be indicative of heart and lung problems, as well as kidney and gastrointestinal issues, it's imperative to get a clear diagnosis of the source of the discomfort.

After taking a full medical history, the doctor will conduct a physical examination and attempt to evaluate both the location and severity of the pain.

The best avenue for accurate diagnosis, however, is the use of imaging tests like X-rays or an MRI. The latter is especially good to find bone spurs or to locate a herniated disc.

X-rays may be taken as part of a myelogram, which involves injecting dye into the spinal column to precisely identify areas of pressure.

If an MRI is not an option for any reason, a CT scan will likely be ordered.

Treating Thoracic Disc Disease

Under the direction of a physical therapist, a program of low-impact aerobic exercise and core strengthening is the first line of treatment for thoracic disc disease. Both walking and bicycling are standard options.

An initial period of complete rest may be ordered, with subsequent modification of activities that seem to worsen the condition.

Over-the-counter non-steroidal anti-inflammatory pain medications are preferred to narcotic drugs, and alternating applications of heat and cold may be helpful. Many patients report significant pain relief and improvement via chiropractic manipulation.

In some instances, epidural injections of steroids are ordered to lower inflammation in the region. All of these approaches should be paired with back-strengthening exercises.

Surgery is typically indicated only when significant bone spurs are present that are compressing the spinal cord and causing neurological symptoms like tingling, numbness, and weakness in the legs.

The goal of the surgery is to remove the compression and may involve the use of rods or plates to limit or stop motion in the problem region. If the diseased disc is removed, a bone graft or other device may be put in its place to facilitate bone fusion and healing.

There are no total disc replacement prosthetics for the thoracic spine like those used in the cervical spine or neck.

Part 2 – Disc Disease by Region

(Thoracic procedures will be discussed in Part 3, which considers Standard Medical Treatments for degenerative disc conditions.)

Lumbar Disc Disease

Although the lumbar region is comprised of only five vertebrae, it is the most likely area of the spine for disc degeneration to be present.

Lumbar disc disease with attendant lower back pain is the second most common reason patients see their primary care physicians, and the fifth most common reason for scheduled appointments with orthopedists.

In the developed world, estimates suggest that 60% to 80% of all adults will experience lumbar disc disease as they age, a condition easily exacerbated by injury and obesity.

Diagnosing Lumbar Disc Disease

Lumbar disc disease carries a range of clear symptoms. It presents with continuous low-grade pain that necessitates only mild palliative measures.

From time to time, however, there will be intense flare ups that are much more problematic, and may increase in frequency as the individual ages.

Symptoms of lower back disc degeneration include:

- Aching pain in the center of the lower back with radiating sensation into the hips and legs.

- Pain that is present for more than six weeks.

- Lower back pain that is more intense when sitting as opposed to standing, walking, or lying down.

- Pain aggravated by prolonged standing, bending forward, or picking up an object.

- More intense pain when twisting, lifting, or bending.

- Numbness and/or tingling in the legs, which can include difficulty walking.

In some cases of collapsed disc, the exiting nerve root may become pinched causing severe, shooting pains in the affected leg.

Your doctor should take an extensive medical history and ask that you describe not just your pain and symptoms, but also your daily activities.

This will include questions about physical positions, overall posture, repetitive movements, amounts lifted, and duration of times standing and sitting.

In a physical exam, your range of motion and muscle strength should also be evaluated along with any localized tenderness. Typically an MRI will be ordered both to pinpoint the location of the diseased disc and to rule out any other potential causes of the discomfort.

Treating Lumbar Disc Disease

For the most part, lumbar disc disease can be treated conservatively without surgery using over-the-counter medications to control pain and inflammation.

Alternating hot and cold packs are a standard strategy for greater comfort. In more severe cases, epidural injections of steroids are also effective.

Surgery is typically only considered if no relief has been achieved after six months, or if the pain is significantly affecting the patient's life.

It's important to identify aggravating activities and to modify or eliminate them from the daily or work routine. Many patients benefit from learning the correct way to lift, as well as how to design more ergonomic working and sleeping spaces.

A program of exercise designed by a physical therapist can facilitate pain relief, improve posture, and strengthen the surrounding muscle structures. Some patients also find working with a chiropractor to be tremendously helpful.

Part 3 – Standard Medical Treatments

Standard medical treatments for degenerative disc disease start with a program of non-operative intervention and only proceed to surgery in the most extreme cases.

Because these problems tend to present as episodic "flare-ups," most treatments focus on pain relief and supportive measures until the acute phase has resolved.

Non-Operative Treatments

The initial response to degenerative disc-related conditions is always conservative. Back surgery should only be considered after all other methods have been tried.

While it is true that the majority of back surgeries are performed with no complications, all the general risks of surgery apply, including, but not limited to:

- a reaction to the anesthesia
- excessive bleeding
- post-operative infections
- the development of blood clots
- heart attack and stroke

In cases of degenerative disc disease, herniation can be recurrent, so a single surgery may not fully resolve the problem. Additionally, there is always a risk of collateral damage leading to weakness, partial or full paralysis, and even greater pain.

If you do consider back surgery, you must understand that the procedures do not always provide significant relief.

Always proceed from a position of informed consent, learning everything you can about any surgery before agreeing to move forward with the operation.

Physical Therapy

Depending on the location of the affected disc, you may have to have access to specific equipment for a program of physical therapy to be helpful.

In many cases, however, the therapist will design a set of exercises specific to your problem and teach you how to perform them correctly at home.

You may find that you will be including many of these stretches in your daily routine, especially if your job involves extended periods of sitting, lifting, or engaging in tasks that can lead to repetitive stress injuries.

A solid program of physical therapy for degenerative disc disease is both therapeutic and preventive in nature.

Cervical Disc Disease Exercises

Exercises designed to help with degenerative cervical disc disease concentrate on stretching and strengthening the neck while improving posture.

The therapist will take initial measurements to determine strength and flexibility that will serve as benchmarks to measure progress.

You will then receive a set of exercises to be performed with supervision and at home that will likely include some variation of:

- Stretches that move the chin to the chest to strengthen the muscles at the back of the neck.

- Slow swivels from side to side.

- Lifting the chin upward in an "eyes to the sky" motion that works on the front of the neck and upper chest area.

- Moving the ear down to the shoulder to stretch and extend the side of the neck. (When performed with guidance, the therapist will place his hand on the head to help direct and deepen this extension.)

When performing neck exercises in the home setting, always apply a headed compress or heating pad to the neck muscles to loosen up the area before stretching the muscle.

At the end of the exercise period, use a cold pack to prevent additional inflammation and take an over-the-counter non-steroidal anti-inflammatory like ibuprofen.

Thoracic Disc Disease Exercises

In cases of thoracic disc disease a physical therapist will conduct movement and strength tests to determine the existing level of flexibility. This will include an analysis of your posture.

Care must be taken not to increase the level of inflammation present, so initial stretches will be geared toward improving blood circulation to optimize healing.

The components of your physical therapy exercise may include any combination of:

- Soft tissue massage including stretching and joint mobilization to improve spinal alignment, flexibility, and range of motion.

- Exercises to strengthen the abdominal muscles to provide better stability and support for the back.

- Retraining to improve posture while standing, sitting, and sleeping. This may include the use of posture aids to support spinal alignment.

Other techniques that may be effective for inflammation and pain in the thoracic region include:

Ultrasound

These treatments are administered with a small wand that directs sonic wave vibrations through the soft tissues to relax muscles tension and improve flexibility.

Ultrasound may also improve the body's ability to produce collagen, which accelerates healing.

Electrical Stimulation

There are two common forms of electrical stimulation for back pain, TENS and IDET. The theory behind each is similar.

Both send electrical stimulation into areas of dense nerve concentration with the intent of disrupting or "scrambling" the nerves' ability to transmit pain signals to the brain.

Radiofrequency Discal Nucleoplasty

This procedure is a newer, similar in nature to electrical stimulation. It uses a probe that directs radio treatment frequencies into the discs to achieve partial decompression for pain relief.

Cold Laser

Cold lasers are a pain management technique based on sending precise wavelengths of light into the tissue in bursts of 30 seconds or more. The level of penetration is approximately 2-5 cm below the skin.

The belief is that the light stimulates processes in the cells that reduce pain, inflammation, and swelling to enhance healing.

Traction

Traction is a much more traditional therapy for back pain that is used by physical therapists and chiropractors. It involves the application of force to gently stretch the soft tissues and increase the shared space between the vertebrae.

There are multiple methods for performing traction therapy, including manual application, positional exercises, or the use of weighted devices.

Pinning down any one series of thoracic exercises or therapies as the most effective is difficult since this is not the most typical region for degenerative disc issues.

Pain in this area may be complicated by other back injuries. Consequently, all physical therapy approaches must be individually tailored. Doing the wrong series of exercises for thoracic disc degeneration will only aggravate the problem.

Part 3 – Standard Medical Treatments
Lumbar Disc Disease Exercises

The lumbar or lower back region is the most common area where disc degeneration symptoms are experienced. Experts are universal in their agreement that exercise is essential to eliminate the painful effects of lower back pain.

A mistake most people make is resting too much when they experience an episode of lower back pain. Generally only a day or two of rest is recommended before actively addressing the acute discomfort.

Low-impact aerobic exercises are the best way to start. Simply walking will help to get the blood flowing to the affected spinal structures to facilitate healing and to relieve pressure on the discs.

Swimming is also an excellent exercise to increase flexibility since your body is fully supported by the buoyancy of the water.

Cycling is also recommended, but only if the seat and handlebars of your bike are well adjusted so as not to aggravate back pain. If you can't ride a regular bike, consider using a recumbent bike at home or at the gym.

Recumbent bikes have chair-like seats with extra cushioning in the lumbar region. You do not have to hunch over the handlebars. Many people prefer this type of bike anyway, since it's easier to read or watch a video while you exercise.

Degenerative Disc Disease Explained P a g e | 47

Working with a physical therapist or a chiropractor, you should also learn a series of back-strengthening exercises including hamstring stretches. Tightness in the hamstrings increases stress on the lower back.

The same ancillary treatments used in thoracic back pain can also be applied to the lumbar region including ultrasound, electrical stimulation, cold laser, and traction.

It is essential, however, that you learn as much as you can about ergonomics and the correct positioning of the body not just for lifting, but also for all daily motions. Even sitting in a poorly adjusted chair with no lumbar support can significantly increase lower back pain.

Often people with disc degeneration in the lower back will need to invest in ergonomically designed furniture for their homes and offices, and buy better mattresses and pillows.

Poor posture is not just limited to how we sit or stand. Stresses on the back at night can make getting up in the morning an agony of stiff muscles and shooting lower back pains.

With the help of your physical therapist, evaluate all the things you do in your life, including recreational activities that may be aggravating your condition. Modifying or eliminating those movements is key to managing lumbar disc disease symptoms.

Common Prescribed Medications

For the most part you should be able to control pain from degenerative disc disease, regardless of location, with over-the-counter non-steroidal pain medicines like:

- aspirin
- ibuprofen
- naproxen

If these prove ineffective, your doctor may prescribe any of the following medications:

- celecoxib
- diclofenac
- diflunisal
- etodolac
- fenoprofen
- flurbiprofen
- indomethacin
- keoprofen
- ketorolac
- meloxicam
- nabumetone
- oxaprozin
- piroxicam
- salsalate
- sulindac
- tolmetin

Due to their addictive qualities, the use of narcotic painkillers should be avoided in all but the most extreme cases.

Some of the most commonly used medications of this genre for back pain include:

- codeine
- fentanyl
- hydrocodone
- hydromorphone
- meperidine
- methadone
- morphine
- oxycodone

Before agreeing to take any medication, it is imperative that you discuss all possible side effects with your doctor and explore potential interactions with other drugs you are taking.

Have this same conversation with your pharmacist, who may well understand drug interactions better than your physician!

It also pays to do your own research online so you can ask the right questions. Never take a prescription medication of any kind until you are absolutely comfortable with the decision to use the drug.

Pay attention to all safety precautions about driving and operating machinery while using painkillers. Many of these drugs cause drowsiness and impair judgment.

Never drink alcoholic beverages while using painkillers. Not only is the interaction of the alcohol with the medication dangerous, the use of alcohol actually intensifies back pain.

Alcohol effects nerve transmissions in the body, and also has a depressant effect on your mood after the "buzz" has worn off.

Depression is a significant hurdle in living with chronic pain. Drinking will only make coping with your condition harder.

Epidural Steroid Injections

Epidural injections paired with some type of numbing agents are intended to both relieve back pain and to decrease inflammation.

The shots do not work uniformly for all patients, but they are particularly well suited to the sharp pains typical of nerve damage in the neck and lower back.

This "radiculopathy" typically originates at the point at which a nerve exits the spine. Epidural injections target the epidural space, the area lying between the spine's protective covering and the vertebrae themselves.

Epidural injections are also useful in cases of spinal stenosis, which is a narrowing of the spinal canal causing compression of the spinal cord or its adjacent nerve structures.

Typically an epidural is performed as an out-patient procedure at a doctor's office by an anesthesiologist or radiologist.

The procedure is a simple one, involving the guided insertion of the needle using a live X-ray or fluoroscope. This allows the doctor to correctly position the needle for the placement of the corticosteroid medication.

Since a numbing medication is used first, the injection is not usually painful, although the site may be tender for a few days afterwards.

Heat and Cold Therapy

As an aspect of all kinds of back therapy, alternating applications of heat and cold are a standard intervention. Some people swear by this approach, while others say heat and cold only makes them feel worse.

Since you should never do anything that aggravates pain in any area of the spine, you will have to judge for yourself the effectiveness of any of these recommendations.

Heat and Moist Heat

Moist heat for 15 to 20 minutes can be a great way to loosen up tight areas of the back and relieve pain. The application may be as simple as standing under a hot shower or soaking in a bath.

Dry heat can be administered in a variety of ways, including "all-day" hot liniment patches. If you use a heating pad, another popular method, take care not to fall asleep using the device.

Set a timer for 20 minutes to make sure you do not burn your skin. Never use a heating pad on the highest setting. Medium or low will produce plenty of radiating warmth.

Ice Packs

Many people who are willing to use heat for back pain find the application of ice packs excruciating. The cold can relieve pain and bring down swelling and inflammation, but some people find the cold sensation itself too uncomfortable.

Recommended methods for applying cold treatments include:

Iced Towels

Wet a towel with cold water and wring it out until the material is barely damp. Fold the towel into a comfortable

pad and place it in a plastic back in the freezer for 15 minutes. Remove the towel and apply it to the painful area.
Bags of Ice

Place ice in a plastic bag and add just enough water to cover the cubes. Squeeze all the air out of the bag, sealing it tightly. Wrap the bag in a wet towel and apply it to your back.

Slush Packs

Mix 3 parts water to 1 part rubbing alcohol in the desired amount inside a plastic freezer back. Seal the bag tightly and put in the freezer until it turns into "slush."

This method allows the bag to conform to the shape of your body and the "slush" can be refrozen multiple times so long as the bag remains intact.

Bag of Vegetables

A bag of frozen vegetables is another take on the slush pack idea. The bag will also conform in shape to the affected area of the body, especially if you use something like frozen corn or peas.

If none of these methods are comfortable or work for you, simply take ice cubes and rub them over the painful area for 3-5 minutes. Some people find this is more tolerable since they can remove the ice for several seconds at a time.

Part 3 – Standard Medical Treatments

When using ice for pain management, apply the treatment at least 3 times a day for 72 hours at a minimum duration of 10-15 minutes.

Surgical Treatment Options

Although the standard procedures to address degenerative disc disease in the back are fusions and/or disc replacements, these procedures will be discussed individually by spinal region since the surgeries carry unique precautions and potential complications dependent on location.

It should be noted, however, that back surgery is rarely indicated in cases of degenerative disc disease and should be the course of last resort. All back surgeries are serious in nature and result in fairly lengthy periods of recuperation.

Since these procedures involve not only healing of the tissues at the site of the incision, but bone healing as well, many preoperative precautions are necessary, in particular stopping smoking and avoiding tobacco use during post-surgical recovery.

Cervical Disc Procedures

The cervical or neck region of the spine is highly prone to the effects of degenerative disc disease. This part of the spinal column not only supports the weight of the head, but is in constant motion as we go about our daily lives, thus experiencing a great deal of wear and tear.

In almost all cases, conservative treatment is recommended over surgery until the cervical problem effects quality of life to an unacceptable degree including the presence of chronic pain.

Anterior Cervical Discectomy and Fusion

Disc fusion surgery seeks to stop the motion of the affected vertebral segment, which means the entire disc is taken out and replaced by a bone graft held in place by screws, an interbody cage, or a supportive plate for stability.

In time, the body's own ability to produce bone to heal fractures takes over, and the intervertebral space becomes fused.

The most generally selected option is to fuse one vertebrae, a "one-level" fusion, but in some rare cases a two-level fusion may be considered.

This surgery returns a 90% success rate in resolving pain, but there is always a danger of a bone graft refusing to grow, a condition called a "non-union." This is less likely in cases where the patient donates the bone graft from another location, typically the pelvis.

Self-donation does mean the patient will be healing from two surgical sites, but this avenue greatly increases the overall chance of the fusion being successful. Non-unions are more likely in cases where cadaver bone from a bone bank is utilized.

It should also be noted that the segments above and below the graft that remain mobile will now absorb the bulk of the daily strain placed on the neck.

In approximately 25% of cases, these discs will show signs of painful degeneration within 10 years, a development termed "adjacent-segment degeneration."

Cervical Disc Replacement

The replacement of degenerated cervical discs with prosthetic or artificial discs is intended to circumvent the problem of non-union of grafts.

Additionally, a prosthetic disc implant will preserve range of motion in the neck and help to avoid future instances of adjacent-segment degeneration.

Artificial discs are used most commonly in the neck. Two types of these implants are currently used. The first is an arrangement of two endplates with an intervening layer of a low friction material to facilitate motion.

These device designs include:

Metal and Polyethylene

Artificial discs made of metal and polyethylene disc replacements are similar to the devices used in hip and knee replacement surgeries.

Metal and Polyurethane

Artificial discs made of metal and polyurethane are identical in design to those made with polyethylene, but the polyurethane is considered to be a softer material.

A second option is a metal-on-metal design that also preserves motion. Both are considered safe for implantation in the cervical region, and undoubtedly are the forerunners of more refined medical devices to come.

Thoracic Disc Procedures

The most commonly surgical procedure in the thoracic region of the spine is designed to address herniated discs. Traditionally, the standard operation was a posterior laminectomy.

Laminectomy

During a laminectomy, the surgeon may remove bone spurs or other segments of bone or ligaments in an effort to relieve pressure on spinal nerves and the discs themselves.

The incision, which is made on the posterior side of the body, is typically extensive. Overall, the procedure tends to destabilize the spine, so that a spinal fusion may have to be performed at the same time or in a subsequent surgery.

An additional limitation of using a laminectomy is that the procedure does not allow access to the central component of the herniated disc itself.

Thoracotomy

A thoracotomy takes a frontal approach to reach the thoracic spine through the chest cavity. While this sounds massively invasive, some spinal centers now perform the surgery as Video Assisted Thoracic Surgery (VATS).

Small incisions allow the insertion of video scopes to guide the surgeon's work. This lets the surgeon access discs that are centrally or centro-laterally herniated.

Costotransversectomy

A costotransversectomy procedure allows work to be performed on laterally herniated thoracic discs from the back and side. A rib is removed, as is the transverse process, which is a small spinal bone.

Via this method, the surgeon can gain access to the disc space, again without the overall de-stabilization seen in the older laminectomy.

Lumbar Disc Procedures

The most typical procedure performed on patients with severe pain due to degenerative disc disease in the lumbar region is a disc fusion.

Disc replacement surgery is also an option, but the procedure is highly complicated in this region and is not widely performed.

Lumbar Disc Fusion

The incision in lumbar disc fusion surgery may be through the abdomen and/or the back. The goal of the procedure is to stop or to stabilize the motion of a degenerated disc that is causing pain and that has not responded to less conservative treatments.

By using some type of hardware like pedicle screws, an interbody cage, spacers, or a structural bone graft, the affected segment of the spine is immobilized.

The affected disc is removed and replaced with a bone graft from the patient's own pelvis or with cadaver bone from a bone bank.

The body's natural mechanism for healing fractures is thus stimulated, and that portion of the spine becomes fused.

Artificial Disc Replacement

Artificial disc replacement is a newer procedure and is sometimes called "total disc replacement." It involves multiple steps:

- An incision is made in the lower wall of the abdomen.
- The abdominal muscles or "six pack" are dissected.

- The abdominal organs are moved to the side.

- The degenerated disc is removed.

- The proper height of the disc space is restored.

- Any adjacent contracted ligaments are released.

- An artificial disc implant is inserted.

This surgery has been performed in Europe for a number of years, and has been available in the U.S. since 2004. In the U.S. it is more commonly performed as a cervical or neck procedure due to the complexity of entering the spinal region via the abdomen, but the thoracic version of the procedure is becoming more common.

Part 4 – Alternative Treatments and Self-Care

Since degenerative disc disease and the pain it causes are typically episodic, patients can avail themselves of a range of techniques to deal with a flare up, and to stave off future incidents.

Exercise for Healing and Prevention

Exercise is important to facilitate healing of back problems and to prevent the pain from returning. A recommended regimen includes gentle, low impact aerobic exercises that are designed to strengthen and stretch the back.

Exercise facilitates the movement of nutrients through the spinal structures. As we exercise, the intervertebral discs swell with water, which is then squeezed back out allowing the discs and other spinal structures to exchange nutrients. This process speeds up healing.

In people who do not exercise, this efficient exchange does not occur, and the risk of developing back problems is higher. Walking, cycling, swimming, and yoga are all considered good forms of exercise to strengthen the back.

Custom Braces

Some people find relief from wearing back braces custom fitted to their bodies that limit painful motion and support the spinal structure during a flare up of back pain.

Part 4 – Alternative Treatments and Self-Care

Your primary care physician may even recommend that you be fitted for such a brace in order to decrease the need for painkillers, including over-the-counter medications that can cause gastrointestinal distress.

Narcotic painkillers carry the added risk of addiction when used over the long term, so secondary supportive and self-care measures are routinely explored to avoid this occurrence.

Your doctor will refer you to a facility that constructs braces and orthotics. During a consultation, you will be measured for the device, and depending on the model chosen, a mold may be made of your back to exactly replicate the curve of your spine.

(Typically health insurance policies will cover the cost of custom braces when they are prescribed by a doctor.)

The downside of wearing a custom brace is that the devices, even when custom fitted, are generally uncomfortable when in place for several hours, especially during hot weather.

Chiropractic Treatments

Chiropractic treatment for degenerative disc disease is a comprehensive approach involving a detailed medical history to determine precise restrictions on motion and the nature of any injuries suffered to the back.

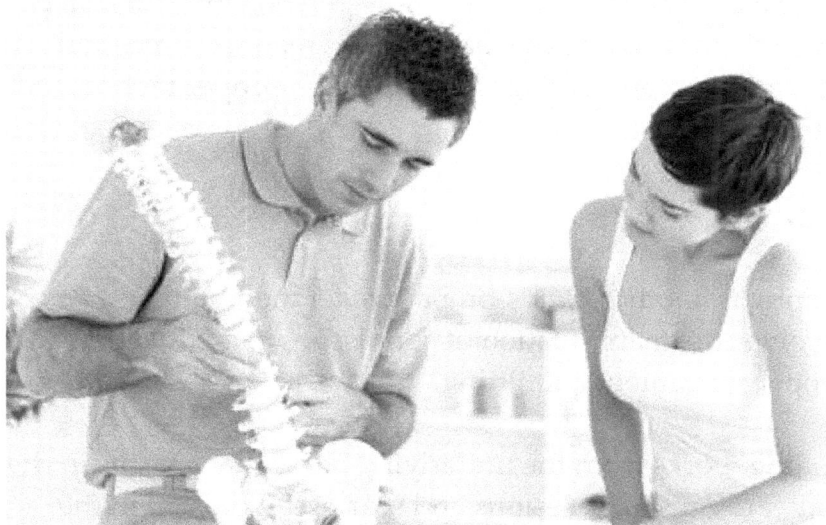

You will be asked to walk and make other motions while the chiropractor observes your posture and range of motion. Imaging tests like X-rays or an MRI may also be useful.

The goal of chiropractic treatment is to improve the spine's mobility through better joint function and decreased levels of inflammation.

Spinal manipulation techniques will be applied along with therapeutic massage, stretching and resistance work, and trigger point pressure techniques.

Both interferential electrical stimulation of the muscles and ultrasound are useful to stimulate blood flow, decrease spasms, and heal inflammation.

Since chiropractors treat the whole person, you will also be given dietary advice as well as tips to manage stress and education on preventing injury through proper motion and lifting.

Rolfing

Rolfing is another hands-on pain relief method that involves the manipulation of soft tissues and education on proper movement and lifting.

Rolfing works from the underlying belief that spasms in the body are caused by lesions and scar tissue present in the muscles, fascia, and tendons.

These abnormal structures inhibit our range of motion and cause pain. If they can be released, flexibility will increase and pain will decrease.

By releasing this scar tissue through manipulation, the range of motion is restored. Although Rolfing, like chiropractic manipulation, will not "heal" a degenerated disc, the technique can build a better muscular support system in the affected area and decrease inflammation.

Also, Rolfing emphasizes the necessity of good posture, so clients frequently report that they stand straighter and even taller after a course of treatments.

Poor posture is a major contributor to back pain, making Rolfing an attractive alternative treatment approach.

Acupuncture

As a mainstay of traditional Chinese medicine, acupuncture treatments are predicated on the belief that the body's energy force, the "chi," can be blocked leading to pain and illness. Freeing the flow of the chi along channels called meridians relieves the pain and restores health.

The needles used in treatments are almost as thin as a single strand of human hair. Multiple needles will be inserted at pre-mapped points on the meridians and left in place for 20-40 minutes.

Western researchers believe that the action of the needles releases neurotransmitters like serotonin or endorphins that speed up the healing process.

Although the precise effect of acupuncture is not clearly understood, many people with degenerative disc disease report significantly lower pain levels after a course of acupuncture treatment.

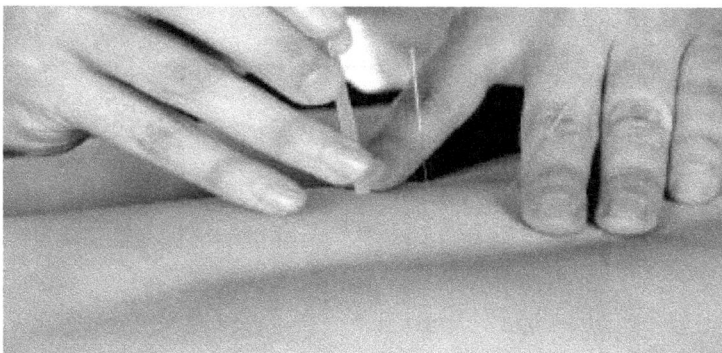

Magnets

Magnet therapy works on assumptions similar to those held in acupuncture that pain can be relieved by altering the energy flow at key points in the body.

These products are widely available in a variety of forms, from single magnets affixed to adhesive patches, to multiple magnets incorporated in braces and wraps.

Magnets are sold in different strengths, with those "rated" for pain relief being 300 to 5000 gauss. There is no clear scientific proof that magnets work, but a wide body of first-person accounts support the therapy.

Since magnet use can be dangerous for people with pacemakers, insulin pumps, or similar medical devices, always consult with your primary physician before trying any of these products.

Meditation

There are many meditative disciplines from mindfulness to transcendental meditation. Some involve clearing the mind of any thought while others call for repetition of a mantra.

Special poses may be required, or simply sitting in a chair with your feet flat on the floor. Music may be playing in the background, or the goal may be complete silence. Time required ranges from 15 minutes to an hour.

The goal, however, is the same in all cases — stress relief and a greater awareness of the body / mind connection. Although some religions incorporate meditative practices, meditation itself is not a religion.

When used in cases of degenerative disc disease and back pain, mediation is largely a pain control technique, and a way to prevent tension from building up in the back muscles.

Scientifically verifiable benefits of meditation include:

- a stronger immune system
- improved digestion
- greater emotional balance
- lower blood pressure
- lowered levels of bodily inflammation

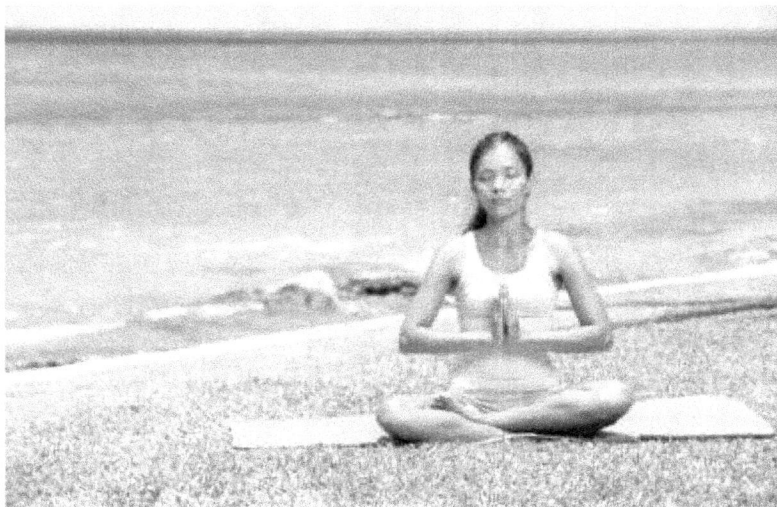

Mediation is generally recommended as a companion approach with standard and alternative treatments for chronic back pain.

Ergonomic Furniture

Ergonomic furniture like desk chairs and easy chairs have been designed specifically to support the spine and to improve resting posture.

Many of us slump in overly soft chairs or work for long hours in torturous desk chairs that are incorrectly adjusted for our height and weight.

Although ergonomic furniture is more expensive, it is often a necessary expedient to prevent constant aggravation of the symptoms of degenerative disc disease, especially of the lower back.

Herbal Remedies

With any use of herbs to treat a health condition, it's always wise to check with your doctor or pharmacist to make sure the items used will not conflict with your prescription medications.

The herbs most often recommended to combat back problems have anti-inflammatory and analgesic properties. The most popular are:

- Devil's Claw, an herb indigenous to South Africa, is traditionally used as treatment for arthritis and gastrointestinal distress. It is an anti-inflammatory agent and is available in capsule form.

- White Willow Bark was a precursor to the development of aspirin. Many people who find synthetic aspirin to be a gastrointestinal irritant tolerate White Willow Bark quite well, and get a similar anti-inflammatory and pain relieving effect from the supplement.

- SAMe or S-adenosylmethionine works to support age-related degenerative conditions like osteoarthritis and degenerative disc disease. It is naturally present in the human body, but people who have insufficient levels of the chemical may be more susceptible to pain and depression.

Alternative Therapies in Combination

While it is not safe to mix pain medications to treat back and neck pain from degenerative disc disease, you can try various combinations of these alternative treatments to seek maximum relief.

Meditation is recommended as a corollary treatment to almost any kind of therapy for back problems, and acupuncture is also often used in combination with chiropractic manipulation of Rolfing.

When using herbal remedies, it is best to make sure that the supplements will not conflict with prescription medications or with one another, but it is still possible to take multiple supplements at once.

Many people are drawn to alternative self-care for the simple reason that it makes them feel as if they are actively working to resolve their back pain.

Special Section – Coping with Chronic Pain

In most cases the pain associated with degenerative disc disease is episodic, presenting in brief, acute flare ups. These episodes may go on for years, however, so it's still important to master techniques for coping with chronic pain.

Stress Reduction

Most of the techniques discussed here have a central goal of releasing stress and counteracting negative feelings that may range from anger and impatience to anxiety, sadness, frustration, and depression.

No two people will respond equally to the same relaxation techniques, so don't give up. If a technique like guided imagery doesn't let you craft a mental escape, but beautiful music calms your mind and relaxes your body, then stock up on CDs and download MP3s to your heart's content!

Whatever works, use it!

Some Things That Don't Work

Having a stiff drink -- or several -- when you're in pain may seem like a good idea, or even a culturally acceptable way to take the edge off. The physiological truth, however, is that alcohol has a depressive effect on your mood, it inhibits nerve activity in the body, slows healing, and interferes with sleep.

None of those things are going to help you really manage your pain.

Endorphins, Natural Drug of Choice

Instead of using alcohol, find some exercise you can do -- even just taking a walk -- to get your body's own feel good drugs, endorphins pumping. Endorphins are peptides secreted by the brain that have an analgesic effect because they stimulate opiate receptors in the body.

That runner's high? That notion of "hitting the wall" and then feeling better? It's real. You don't have to run a marathon to get a "hit" of endorphins. For most people a nice brisk walk in the fresh air will do the same thing.

If you're not the outdoors type? Get on the treadmill or even a stationary bike. You will feel better afterwards.

Practice Deep Breathing

Holding your breath or breathing very shallowly is a common reaction to pain. This causes a build-up of tension, tightening the muscles of the body and making the pain worse. Deep breathing is a good technique to release that tension. An added benefit is increased blood flow and oxygenation, which facilities healing.

Meditation experts recommend visualizing a balloon in the stomach. As you breathe in, fill the balloon. Put your hands on your stomach so you can feel the air moving into the balloon. Exhale just as deeply, deflating the balloon just as you filled it.

You can practice this technique anywhere, but at least once or twice a day, try to find a quiet spot and really get comfortable. Use your deep breathing as a form of meditation to settle your thoughts and take a break for a few minutes.

Don't Concentrate on the Pain

The more you think of your pain, the more you will hurt. It's crucial to find some activity that completely absorbs your mind. Concentration is a powerful pain reliever, especially when you're doing something you enjoy. If you don't have a hobby or an all-consuming project, find one!

Keep a Pain Journal

While the suggestion to keep a pain journal may seem to contradict the advice not to focus exclusively on the pain, it's important to understand all kinds of situations that make your pain worse.

In the case of a bad back, this may be how you're sitting, or even the weight of your briefcase in your hand on the way to the office.

It may be more illuminating, however, when you realize that your pain is worse after a tense conversation with your boss because you're tense. That's when some deep breathing is in order.

Tracking your pain allows you to find your triggers and either head them off in advance, or be prepared to deal with them in the aftermath.

Be Kind to Yourself

Some days will be better than others. There will be times when you need the painkillers, or when staying on the heating pad is all you want to do. It's okay to indulge those feelings for a day or two, but you can rest a bad back too much and wind up with an even more debilitated state.

It's okay to be patient with yourself and kind, but realize that living with chronic pain is an active process that involves both the mind and the body.

Epidural injections paired with some type of numbing agents are intended to both relieve back pain and to decrease inflammation.

The shots do not work uniformly for all patients, but they are particularly well suited to the sharp pains typical of nerve damage in the neck and lower back.

This "radiculopathy" typically originates at the point at which a nerve exits the spine. Epidural injections target the epidural space, the area lying between the spine's protective covering and the vertebrae themselves.

Epidural injections are also useful in cases of spinal stenosis, which is a narrowing of the spinal canal causing compression of the spinal cord or its adjacent nerve structures.

Typically an epidural is performed as an out-patient procedure at a doctor's office by an anesthesiologist or radiologist.

The procedure is a simple one, involving the guided insertion of the needle using a live X-ray or fluoroscope. This allows the doctor to correctly position the needle for the placement of the corticosteroid medication.

Since a numbing medication is used first, the injection is not usually painful, although the site may be tender for a few days afterwards.

Part 5 – Nutrition and Spinal Health

Eating a healthy diet with a good variety of vitamins and nutrients provides a broad spectrum of benefits that contribute to overall wellbeing.

Obviously diet is integral in maintaining an optimal weight, with obesity significantly contributing to back problems associated with degenerative disc disease.

You may be surprised to learn, however, that nutrition offers some highly specific benefits for spinal health in particular.

Hydration and Disc Health

Most people in the developed world live in a state of low-level, chronic dehydration even though they have access to plentiful supplies of clean drinking water. Poor hydration is linked to:

- chronic fatigue
- constipation and other digestive disorders
- urinary tract infections
- difficulty in regulating blood pressure
- respiratory conditions
- obesity
- skin conditions including eczema
- high cholesterol

The human body is made up of 60-70% water, which is essential for the transport of nutrients to all the major organs, as well as for the removal of wastes.

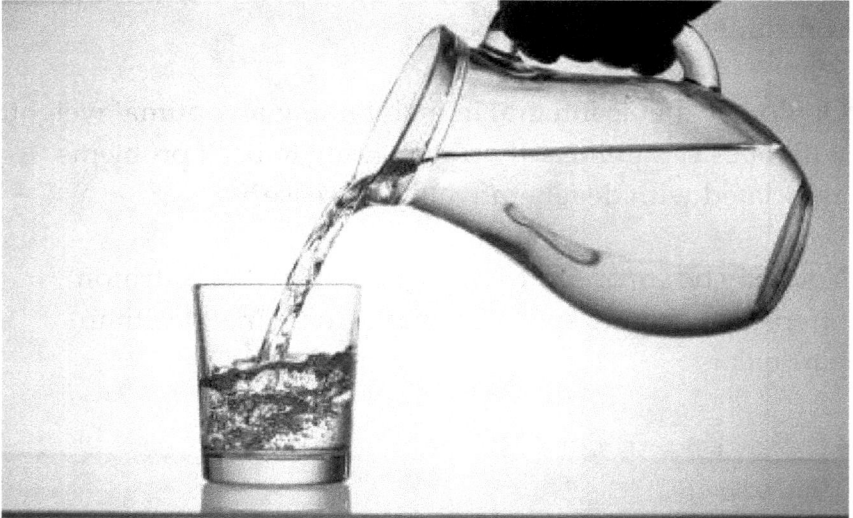

A lesser known fact, however, is the role hydration plays in protecting the body's joints and ensuring proper spinal function. The intervertebral discs are, themselves, largely made of water. At birth, the discs are 80% water, but that level decreases with age.

During day-to-day activities the force of gravity combined with the pressure of movement and exercise slowly squeezes water out of the discs.

At night, the discs relax and rehydrate. Without adequate levels of water in the body to draw on, the rehydration cannot occur, or is less efficient.

The standard recommendations for daily water consumption by gender are:

- Men, 6.3 pints / 3 liters per day
- Women, 4.6 pints / 2.2 liters

This translates to roughly 8 "large glasses" in common understanding, but in general, always err on the side of more.

Back Pain and Obesity

A well-balanced diet will help to control weight gain and prevent obesity. Excessive abdominal fat adds to back problems by straining the muscles and ligaments that support the spine.

The spinal joints are already vulnerable to the wear and tear of daily living, a condition worsened by a weakening of the body's supportive structures. If inflammation is also present in the body, pain is the inevitable result.

Inflammation and Back Pain

In the most simplistic definition, inflammation is the body's response to injury and infection, a defensive release of immune cells that go on high alert through a flood of increased blood flow.

This system serves us well when a true threat is being posed, but poor nutrition can lead to chronic inflammation, a situation in which the defensive response is inappropriately triggered.

Some foods that contribute to inflammation include:

- Items high in trans fats that damage the lining of the blood vessels.

- Foods like white bread and pasta that are made from refined grains.

- Excessive amounts of animal fats from red meat.

- Alcoholic beverages.

- Foods rich in Omega-6 fatty acids. (Note that Omega-3 fatty acids combat inflammation, so the two should always be kept in balance.)

- Milk.

- Foods that contain monosodium glutamate (MSG).

- Foods that contain gluten.

Inflammation in the joints of the spine leads to a loss of the cellular framework that holds the bones and connective tissues together.

Some people with low levels of inflammation in their bodies can have degenerative disc disease and experience no pain. However, when inflammation is present, the sensation of pain is heightened.

The inflammation causes the growth of new blood and nerve cells in and around the cartilage of the joint or disc. The increased tissue activity and swelling makes the new nerves highly sensitive.

The first key in stopping the pain is relieving the inflammation. Over the long-term, a diet that concentrates on lowering or eliminating inflammation can prevent a recurrence of the back pain, even though the disc degeneration is still present.

Avoid Smoking, Reduce Alcohol Consumption

After poor hydration, some of the most serious insults to spinal health result from the use of tobacco and alcohol.

While the respiratory damage wrought by alcohol is well known, most people don't understand that smoking damages the vascular structures of the joints and intervertebral discs.

As those structures weaken over time due to decreased blood flow and increased inflammation, pain levels increase. Studies have proven a high correlation between painful lumbar disc disease and tobacco use.

Additionally, nicotine inhibits bone growth. This is why patients who are facing spinal fusion surgery are asked to stop smoking well in advance of the procedure, and are urged not to resume smoking afterward. Failure to do either of these things can seriously imperil their chances of a full and successful recovery.

Alcohol acts as a depressant. People with chronic back pain who drink to excess will be less able to cope with their condition because the alcohol will further lower their already depressed mood.

Additionally, the sugar in alcohol has no dietary value, and thus contributes to weight gain and obesity.

Calcium-Rich Foods Are Essential

Calcium is essential to preserve bone mass in the body, but many elements of the modern diet, which are heavy in phosphoric acid, cause excessive calcium loss in the urine.

These include carbonated soft drinks and caffeinated beverages like coffee. On average, the body loses 6 milligrams of calcium for every 100 milligrams of caffeine taken in.

These dietary concentrations build up much faster than we realize when average caffeine volumes are considered:

- 1 oz. (30 mL) coffee has 40-75 mg of caffeine
- 16 oz. (480 mL) latte has 150 mg of caffeine
- 12 oz. (355 mL) classic cola brand 30-35 mg of caffeine
- 2 oz. (60 mL) energy drink 207 mg of caffeine

It is a misconception however, that drinking cow's milk is one of the best ways to return calcium to your system. While it is true that a cup of milk contains about 300 mg of calcium, humans barely absorb that calcium, and milk actually increases calcium loss in the bones.

Cow's milk is an animal protein. It acidifies the pH level of the body, which prompts our system to trigger a neutralizing agent — calcium.

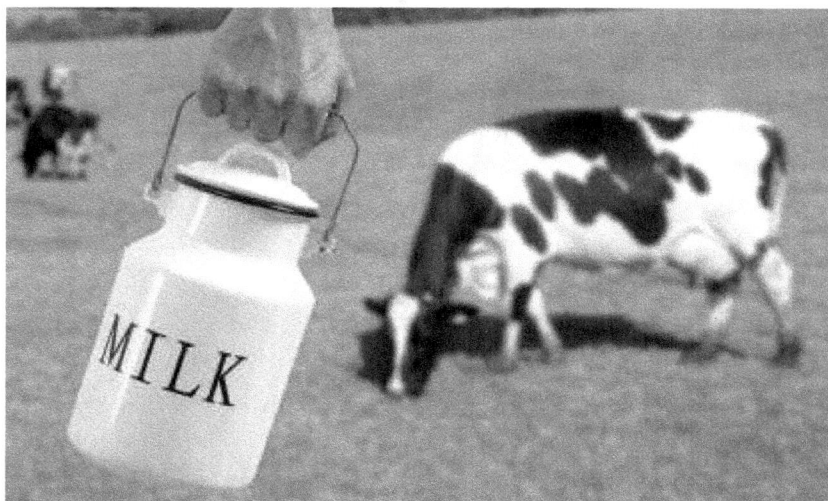

The human body's greatest stores of calcium are found in our bones, so when we drink milk, our body draws calcium out of the bones to counter the acidic effect of that consumption.

When all is said and done, we come away from that healthy glass of milk with less calcium in our bodies, not more – hardly a fact the dairy industry is anxious to see shared on a widespread basis.

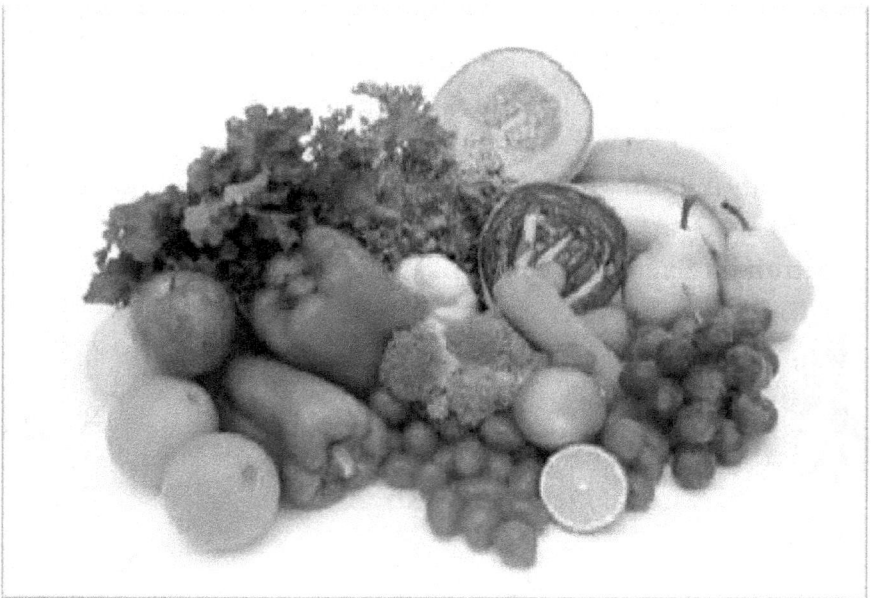

A plant-based diet, however, offers significantly greater amounts of calcium the body can process and store. A cup of steamed kale, for instance has 210 mg of calcium.

A diet that emphasizes plant proteins and starches derived from a variety of fruits and vegetables is far more instrumental in staving off osteoporosis and degenerative disc disease than a diet that includes high amounts of dairy content.

The Vitamin D - Calcium Link

Vitamin D would more appropriately be termed a hormone than a vitamin. It plays a key role in the regulation of human immune function and cell growth, but it is also necessary for the human gut to absorb calcium.

No matter how much calcium you put into your system from healthy sources, it will not be as effective in preventing bone loss and strengthening the connective tissue (collagen) without good Vitamin D levels.

Foods that are rich in Vitamin D include:

- herring
- salmon
- sardines
- tuna
- fortified soy products
- mushrooms
- eggs

If none of these foods are appealing to you, a tablespoon of cod liver oil per day (or a 1000 IU capsule) will be sufficient supplementation to enhance calcium absorption.

Afterword

"Pain in the neck" is such a universally understood concept in Western cultures it's synonymous with having a nagging problem that just won't go way.

For those of us who have actually lived with a pain in our necks, the phrase is pretty ironical. When I was working with a physical therapist for the pain associated with my degenerated cervical disc, I met people with a broad range of spinal problems.

I watched people with serious lower back pain associated with bad lumbar discs struggle to get up out of their chairs. For them, just walking across the room without stooping was a huge achievement.

Frankly, it all put things in perspective for me and I was happy enough to be successfully dealing with my "pain in the neck." The more I realized that my own bad habits were exacerbating the problem, the easier it was for me to wait out my recovery.

I was lucky, after three weeks in physical therapy my range of motion was hugely improved. I still do my exercises at home and if I feel tension at the end of the day I use heat and cold packs. I don't smoke anymore, and I drink more water than I have at any point in my life.

My discs aren't going to suddenly become young again, but I don't have chronic pain and when there is a flare up, I understand what's happened and what I need to do to make it better.

I have a firm belief that information is power, especially in a medical setting. Most of us don't like to go to the doctor, and some people are absolutely terrified at the prospect.

If I had not taken the time to educate myself about the structure of my spine and to learn the words and lingo the doctors were using with me, I don't think I would have been as successful at coping with and largely resolving my neck problems.

My goal in compiling this book was to supply you with the same kind of basic education in overall spinal health. That being said, I'm not a doctor. Nothing here should be taken as a medical recommendation.

I do hope that you will come away better able to listen to and talk with your doctors and therapists to arrive at the best plan for your own spinal health.

As much as we hate to admit it, intervertebral disc degeneration really is a natural consequence of aging, but we don't have to let it turn us into stiff, limited "old folks."

I encourage you to take charge of your spinal health – including taking all the necessary preventive measures – to stay flexible and active.

Afterword

The dime store poster wisdom in this case actually is quite true, "Age is a matter of the mind, and if you don't mind, it doesn't matter."

Anyone can be faced with degenerative disc disease and everyone can find a way to cope with and overcome the problem.

Afterword

Relevant Websites

University of Maryland Medical Center
www.umm.edu/programs/spine/health/guides/degenerative-disc-disease

Dr. Oz
www.doctoroz.com/videos/degenerative-disc-disease-what-you-need-know

Orthogate
www.orthogate.org/patient-education/lumbar-spine/lumbar-degenerative-disc-disease.html

Medical News Today
www.medicalnewstoday.com/articles/266630.php

Science Direct
www.sciencedirect.com/science/article/pii/S0142961213010508

Spine Universe
www.spineuniverse.com/conditions/degenerative-disc-disease

UCLA Neurosurgery
www.neurosurgery.ucla.edu/body.cfm?id=1123&ref=111&action=detail

Wikipedia
www.en.wikipedia.org/wiki/Human_vertebral_column

Relevant Websites

National Center for Biotechnology Information
www.ncbi.nlm.nih.gov/pubmed/10874223

Laser Spine Institute
www.laserspineinstitute.com/back_problems/spinal_anato
my/spine/sacrum/

Youtube
www.youtube.com/watch?v=cdz_qXhgQA8

Google
www.google.com/search?q=Foraminotomy&rlz=1C1TSNO_
enUS492US492&oq=Foraminotomy&aqs=chrome..69i57.372
395j0&sourceid=chrome&espvd=210&ie=UTF-8

Frequently Asked Questions

To really understand all the ways in which intervertebral disc degeneration can cause spinal issues, I recommend you read the entire text.

However, as a quick introduction, the following are some of the most commonly asked questions about disc-related pain in the neck and back.

Does back pain have common causes ?

Not really. In the absence of an obvious injury, back pain can be a frustrating mystery that's all but impossible to pin down. Episodes are most often self-limiting, resolving in a few days or weeks.

In many cases, the root of the problem can be traced to age-related degeneration of the intervertebral discs. Thankfully very few of these problems ever require surgical treatment.

Are their clear risk factors for the development of disc degeneration?

If you are aging, the discs in your spine are deteriorating to some degree. These cushioning structures face constant stress just from the day-to-day movement of our bodies.

Maintaining a healthy weight, refraining from smoking, and staying well hydrated are all good prevented measures to keep all your joints in good shape.

Additionally, it's important to learn how to lift and stand properly, and to maintain good posture. This extends to being concerned about supporting the neck and back while sleeping.

Is anyone at more risk for developing neck or back pain?

Neck and back pain are the bane of working people who use their bodies for hard work with repetitive motion on a daily basis. The pain typically doesn't show up until mid-life, and it actually tends to diminishe after age 70.

The intervertebral discs in the spine get brittle as we age and are more likely to herniate or bulge. There is, however, a somewhat unexpected plus side to this situation.

The discs aren't the only spinal structure to deteriorate. The nerves age as well. The older we get, the less able the spinal nerves are to efficiently transmit pain signals. The underlying structural problems are still there, but they don't hurt as much or at all.

The majority of back and neck problems develop in people in their forties and fifties. The precipitating event is not so much a loss of strength as flexibility.

Most people in mid-life can still lift the same amount of weight, the action just places more stress on the ligaments and muscles than it did one or two decades earlier.

Is there any exercise I can do to strengthen my back?

Absolutely! Get out and walk. The natural action of the human trunk in motion is the best exercise to reduce swelling and to keep the blood flow to the spine at optimal levels.

You can walk as a life-long preventive measure, and as preparation for and recovery from surgery. There's no need to power walk or to pace off huge distances, just get moving.

It doesn't matter if you're outdoors or inside on a treadmill, the benefit of walking is equal in both settings.

I hear the terms "acute" and "chronic" back pain. What's the difference?

The major difference in the two states is the duration. Acute pain flares up suddenly and resolves within six weeks or less. Most back pain falls into this category and can be traced to a specific cause like a fall or picking up something heavy. Chronic back pain continues for at least three months.

What precautions can I take to prevent or decrease back or neck pain?

Monitor your activities to look for triggers for pain in either your back or neck. Modify or eliminate actions that make the pain worse.

If you do something that causes a flare up, use heat and ice therapy along with over-the-counter non-steroidal anti-inflammatories. Consult your doctor if the pain does not resolve in a few days.

Are there any signs or symptoms that would signal a more serious spinal problem?

Truthfully, problems with the spine don't cause a lot of symptoms until they become more advanced. Any or all of the following problems may be warning signs of a spinal issue, or an indication that you've suffered some type of neck or back related injury.

- pain in any part of the back including the neck
- frequent and recurring headaches
- pain in one or both arms or legs
- pain in any joint
- tingling or numbness in one or both arms or legs
- awkward posture you cannot resolve
- insomnia due to pain
- low energy or chronic fatigue

My doctor wants me to have a discogram. What is that?

A discogram is a form of X-ray. A dye is injected into one or more of the discs in your spine before the image is taken. This results in a more sharply contrasted picture so the doctor can more accurately assess the condition of the spine.

My primary care physician diagnosed a bulging disc in my spine. Do I need to get a second opinion from a specialist?

A primary care physician is certainly capable of diagnosing a bulging disc, but you should always feel comfortable with any diagnosis you receive. Never hesitate to seek a second opinion.

In most cases of bulging disc, however, the services of a specialist are only required if you are experiencing numbness, tingling, or weakness in your arms or legs.

What is the difference between a bulging disc and a herniated disc?

There is no difference. In both instances the jelly like substance in the center of an intervertebral disc is pushed outward.

In a bulging disc the material is subjected to force from compression of the disc, whereas a herniated disc occurs when the jelly leaks out through a rupture of the disc's outer shell.

Why do I have pain and weakness in my arm when the problem is in my back?

The spinal column serves as a protective shield for the spinal cord. Up and down the length of the spine, nerves branch off the cord. At the point of exit, a bulging disc or bone spur can press on the nerve, or it can become pinched due to lack of space in cases of spinal stenosis.

Those nerves travel out to the arms and legs in order to send messages to the muscles. When you feel pain or weakness in your arm, the nerve to that region of your body is being affected by an irregularity in your spine.

If I have degenerative disc disease is it a disability?

In the United States, the Social Security Administration technically recognizes degenerative disc disease as the grounds to declare a person disabled, but it's an extremely difficult claim to prove. It is not completely impossible to qualify for benefits on this basis, but it's very hard. In the UK, the condition does not qualify for disability benefits.

Will I need physical therapy for my disc degeneration?

Physical therapy is often recommended as part of a conservative plan to manage the effects of degenerative disc disease.

A guided program of exercise and stretching can help to alleviate pain and strengthen the affected area to prevent future flare-ups.

A specific set of exercises will be formulated for you by a therapist depending on the overall state of your health and the area of your spine being affected by the degeneration.

Frequently Asked Questions

My doctor tells me that I have degenerative disc disease and bone spurs on my spine. Will the pain just continue to get worse?

The word "degenerative" is widely misunderstood in relation to this condition. It doesn't mean your condition will continue to get worse, it means you have the condition because your discs have deteriorated with age.

The same process leads to the formation of bone spurs, which cause pain by limiting your range of motion and pressing on nerves along the spinal column.

Typically, the pain from back problems lessens after age 70 because the nerves in the back also deteriorate. They no longer efficiently process pain signals.

Your problem will still be present, but it may not hurt as much. Still, it is important to maintain your strength and mobility as you age, and to pay attention to good posture.

Frequently Asked Questions

Glossary

A

anterior – A term referring to the front portion of the body often used to describe the relative position of one structure to another.

annulus fibrosus – The ring-like outer portion of an intervertebral disc of the spine composed of a fibrous material.

anterolateral – A locational term describing a structure that is positioned to the front of and to the side of a stipulated point of reference.

arthritis – Arthritis is an inflammatory condition that effects the joints of the human body that presents with swelling and pain resulting in a reduced range of motion.

articular – Of or pertaining to a joint.

B

bone – The hard structures that provide support to the human body classed by the terms long, short, or flat.

bone spur – Growths and rough edges found at the edge of bones. The medical terms for these structures is "osteophytes."

Glossary

bulging disc – When one of the intervertebral discs loses its shape and the soft interior bulges outward due to compression.

C

cartilage – White, thin tissue found where the ends of bones meet at the joints. Cartilage allows for motion of the joints with minimum friction.

cerebrospinal fluid – This protective fluid surrounds the spinal cord and brain, nourishing nerve tissue and removing waste products.

central nervous system – The system of the human body responsible for controlling motor and sensory signals via the brain and spinal cord. The central nervous system works in partnership with the neural network called the peripheral nervous system.

cervical spine – The first seven vertebrae of the spine that make up the neck region of the total structure.

chiropractor – A health care professional who diagnoses and treats problems associated with the muscles and bones of the body, particularly those that present with neck and back pain.

coccyx – The tailbone, which is that region of the spine found below the vertebrae of the sacrum.

Glossary

collapsed disc – A collapsed disc is one of several potential wear and tear injuries of the spine that are degenerative in nature. The aging discs thin to the point of collapsing on themselves, placing pressure on the spinal cord, as well as on the roots of nerves exiting the cord and branching out into the body.

compression – In general terms, compression is the pressing together of two structures. In relation to the spine, compression occurs when a vertebrae loses its natural height and presses against the spinal cord or adjacent nerves.

D

disc – The intervertebral structures of the human spine that separate and cushion the vertebrae. Each disc is composed of an outer fibrous ring called the annulus fibrous and an inner "jelly" known as the nucleus pulposus.

degenerative disc disease– The age-related structural and functional diminishment of the integrity of the intervertebral discs of the spine that effects their ability to cushion and stabilize the total structures.

Discectomy – Surgical removal of part or all of an intervertebral disc.

distal – A positional term indicating that a structure is away from the body's center.

Glossary

E

epidural - In relation to chronic back pain, an epidural refers to an injection of steroids to reduce swelling and inflammation from a degenerated disc and its associated problems. The steroid is placed in the "epidural space," the area located between the spine's protective sheath and the vertebrae.

F

facet – A "joint" at the back of each vertebra to allow motion of the spinal column. For each individual vertebra there are four facets, two superior and two inferior.

foramen - A natural passage or opening in a bone through which other structures like blood vessels pass.

H

herniated disc – A degeneration of an intervertebral disc that occurs when the interior jelly-like material, the "nucleus pulpous" extrudes through tears in the disc's outer covering, the annulus fibrosus.

L

ligament – Bands of connective tissue attached at the end of bones near joints. These flexible, fibrous structures stabilize the joints while serving to attach the bones and allow or prevent given motions.

Glossary

lumbar - The portion of the spine located below the thoracic or chest region and above the sacrum that comprises the lower back and encompasses five individual vertebrae. Basically positioned between the ribs and the pelvis.

M

magnetic resonance imaging (MRI) - A magnetic imaging procedure for scanning the body. This method provides that best images of the spine for diagnostic purposes.

N

nerves – Specialized tissues that conduct messages from the brain and spinal cord throughout the body via electrical impulse and send sensory information back to the brain. This communication network and all its component parts comprises the central nervous system.

neuropathy - Damage to a nerve that may be caused by injury, disease, or the degeneration of adjacent structures. The symptoms include tingling along the path of the nerve, typically in the hands and/or feet. Severe cases can result in the atrophying of muscles and even paralysis.

nucleus pulposus – The jelly like material in the center of an intervertebral disc surrounded by a protective ring called the annulus fibrosus.

O

osteophyte - Outgrowths of bone at the edge of a vertebra or any bony structure commonly called a "spur."

P

physical therapy – Guided treatment with a professional therapist involving exercises to strengthen muscles, increase range of motion, re-learn movements, and rehabilitate damage to the human body.

posture - The position of the human body assumed over time through habit and limitations of physical structure. Poor posture is often a contributing factor to chronic back pain.

S

sacrum – That portion of the spine that is adjacent to the pelvis below the lumbar spine. The sacrum is made up of five vertebrae that are fused so that no intervening discs are present.

spinal stenosis – A condition involving a diminishment of the spinal canal's diameter when new bone forms. The narrowing of the channel can results in direct pressure on either the spinal cord itself or the nerves that branch off it, leading to pain and other physical symptoms.

spinal fusion – The surgical process of permanently joining one or more spinal vertebrae to prevent painful motion associated with degenerative disc disease or other spinal conditions like arthritis.

spinal canal – The vertebrae of the spine form a channel of bone through which the spinal cord passes. The vertebrae protect the spinal cord, while providing openings through which branching nerves may exit the canal and spread into the body.

spinal cord – A long cord comprised of nerve tissue protectively encased in the spinal column that serves as a pathway for nerve impulses to move to and from the brain. The brain, spinal cord, and nerves form the body's central nervous system.

spine – The spine is a column of 33 interconnected vertebrae that begin at the base of the skull and end at the tail bone. This flexible structure is divided into cervical (neck), thoracic (chest), lumbar (lower back), and sacral (pelvic) regions.

T

thinning disc - When an intervertebral disc loses its height due to decreased water content, the disc is said to "thin." This is an aspect of degenerative disc disease, an age-related condition of the spine.

Glossary

thoracic – That portion of the spine located at the level of the chest. These 12 vertebrae, to which the ribs are attached, sit between the cervical (neck) and lumbar (lower back) sections of the spinal column.

V

vertebrae – The 33 cylindrical bones that form the human spinal column and serve to protect the spinal cord, the major neural pathway from the brain to the parts of the body. Note that the singular form of vertebrae is vertebra.

Index

Index

www.ingramcontent.com/pod-product-compliance
Lightning Source LLC
Chambersburg PA
CBHW072237290326
41934CB00008BB/1321

* 9 7 8 0 9 8 9 6 5 8 4 8 5 *